The Anxiety Recovery Journal

The
Anxiety Recovery Journal

Creative Activities to Keep Yourself Well

CARA LISETTE
and *ANNELI ROBERTS*

Foreword by Dr Annie Hickox
Illustrated by Victoria Barron

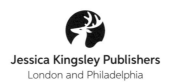

Jessica Kingsley Publishers
London and Philadelphia

First published in Great Britain in 2024 by Jessica Kingsley Publishers
An imprint of John Murray Press

2

A CIP catalogue record for this title is available from the
British Library and the Library of Congress

ISBN 978 1 80501 079 1
eISBN 978 1 80501 080 7

Printed and bound in Great Britain by Bell & Bain Limited

Jessica Kingsley Publishers' policy is to use papers that are natural, renewable and recyclable
products and made from wood grown in sustainable forests. The logging and manufacturing
processes are expected to conform to the environmental regulations of the country of origin.

Jessica Kingsley Publishers
Carmelite House
50 Victoria Embankment
London EC4Y 0DZ

www.jkp.com

John Murray Press
Part of Hodder & Stoughton Ltd
An Hachette Company

Foreword

I first met Cara Lisette and Anneli Roberts on social media a few years ago and was immediately struck by both their honesty about their personal experiences of mental health conditions and their gift of reaching out to others and offering support. As a clinical psychologist, I am always on the lookout for resources for my patients that are accessible and non-judgemental, and I was therefore delighted to learn that Cara and Anneli were working together to create *The Anxiety Recovery Journal,* aimed at anyone who has been experiencing the very real grip of fear and self-doubt that anxiety so often brings.

The authors have created a very readable and practical book, in which they use everyday language to express complex ideas in a non-clinical, validating and encouraging style. This book is not a didactic 'how to...' manual. On the contrary, it is distinctive because of its flexible and individual approach, sensitively encouraging readers to reflect on their own individual needs and to tailor the journal to their own circumstances, and to think, feel and explore factors that may contribute to and maintain anxiety.

Perhaps the most special aspect of *The Anxiety Recovery Journal* is the combined perspective of the two authors: Cara Lisette, a CBT therapist who has lived experience of mental health conditions, and Anneli Roberts, a mental health advocate with firsthand experience of anxiety. Together, their knowledge and experience set this book apart from many others by offering real-life content for anyone suffering from anxiety, whether on its own or co-occurring with another mental health condition. This also gives the book a tangible and personal quality where the reader can feel that the authors have 'tried and tested' the exercises provided.

As a clinician, I particularly enjoyed seeing how the authors translate well-established evidence-based practices into ordinary language. By doing so, they have created a resource which is both deceptively easy to read while also containing substantial components – including thinking errors, behavioural experiments and goal setting – derived from clinical research and practice. These principles are gracefully interweaved with creative exercises and interests such as cooking, drawing and so on, which allow it to be a very personalized experience for the reader.

I anticipate that *The Anxiety Recovery Journal* will be welcomed by the mental health community, both service users and mental health professionals. It will be an extremely valuable adjunct to formal psychological therapy as well as a 'standalone' book that readers can use independently outside of the therapeutic context.

Dr Annie Hickox
Consultant Clinical Psychologist

Hello, reader!

Welcome to your anxiety recovery journal. Throughout this book there are a number of exercises to help you to explore your experiences of anxiety and motivate you to start challenging it, so that one day it may be less of a feature in your life.

We have used our knowledge, both through Cara's clinical and personal experiences as a trained therapist with mental health difficulties and Anneli's lived experience of generalized anxiety disorder, to help create a variety of different exercises which are designed to help you to tap into your creative side and take control of your anxiety.

This is your book to use as you choose: you can write in it, draw in it, decorate it. Creativity is an excellent outlet, and we hope you find that some of these prompts bring you closer to your goals.

This journal is not a replacement for therapy, but a tool to help you learn more about your experience of anxiety and different strategies that may help you.

Keep fighting. There is so much more to life than anxiety, and you deserve to experience it.

Lots of love, Cara and Anneli

A note from Anneli

Hello! I'm Anneli. Thank you so much for picking up this journal. I truly hope that it helps you better understand your anxiety, as well as helping you identify the things that make you feel both better and worse.

I have generalized anxiety disorder and have been living with panic attacks since I was a teenager. Over the years, I've developed a lot of helpful coping strategies and techniques that help me to manage my anxiety day to day, and many of those are reflected in the way we've put this journal together. I want this book to be something that you can turn to when you really need it. A place where you can write down some of the thoughts that are bothering you and stop them from bouncing around your head.

Well done for acquiring this book. You've taken a big step in just acknowledging that you need it and want to make space to tackle your anxiety. As a stranger, I'm proud of you for doing that. Now get yourself a brew and get stuck in. Encouragement and love!

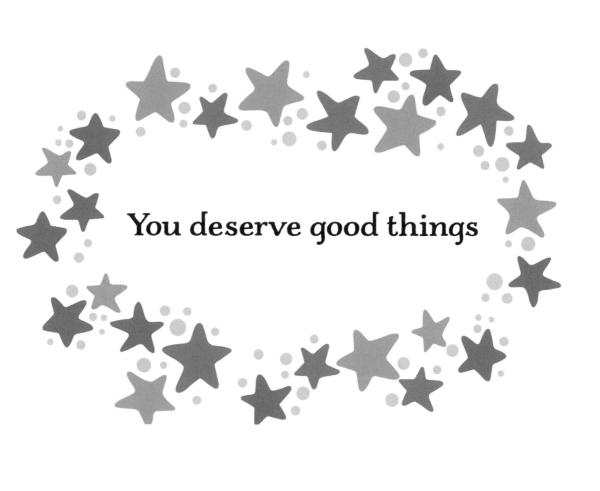

You deserve good things

What is anxiety?

Anxiety is a normal and healthy emotion to feel when we are experiencing times of stress or change. It's our body's response to feeling under threat, and most people will experience anxiety at various times in their life, such as around exams, public speaking, job interviews and more.

Anxiety is often a full-body experience, affecting how we think, feel and behave, and for many people is short lived and situational.

However, for some people anxiety can become a problematic emotion. If you notice your anxiety is impacting your life to the degree where it's disrupting your day-to-day activities, your relationships and your wellbeing, it might be considered a mental health problem that needs additional work to overcome.

You might notice that your anxiety feels disproportionate, difficult to control and long lasting. The good news is, many people who experience these difficulties are able to overcome them and reduce the impact that anxiety has on their life.

My recovery goals

Goal setting can be a really important way of motivating us to make changes, some of which can feel difficult. Thinking about ways your future could be different and things you'd like to do and achieve can provide focus and help you to remember what is important. It's useful to include short-, medium- and long-term goals, and to make sure these feel realistic and achievable. Think about the time frame you'd like to have completed them in so you can keep track of your progress. Let's set some goals. What would you like to achieve, and by when?

1. ....
   ....

2. ....
   ....

3. ....
   ....

4. ....
   ....

5. ....
   ....

6. ....
   ....

7. ....
   ....

8. ....
   ....

9. ....
   ....

10. ....
    ....

My reasons to overcome my anxiety

1. ....
   ....

2. ....
   ....

3. ....
   ....

4. ....
   ....

5. ....
   ....

6. ....
   ....

7. ....
   ....

8. ....
   ....

9. ....
   ....

10. ....
    ....

Helpful mantras

I own my recovery journey and I can move at my own pace

I trust myself. I can handle whatever comes my way

I am responsible enough to keep myself safe
and brave enough to ask for help

Having a bad day does not undo all the progress I have made

Every day I learn a little more about
myself, and I learn to cope better

I am an amazing person, and I deserve an amazing future

I work hard, and I deserve to rest

I have done this before, and I can do it again

I am learning how to be in the present

I did not choose anxiety, but I do choose recovery

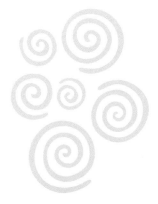

Quotes, lyrics and phrases that inspire me

Quote jars

Quote jars can be a really helpful way to start the day and keep you motivated. Try writing down on pieces of paper some of the mantras from this book and some of the quotes and lyrics that inspire you personally, then fold them up and put them in a jar. You can take one out every morning, or just whenever you feel like you need a boost.

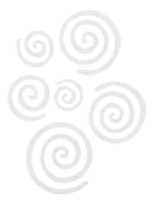

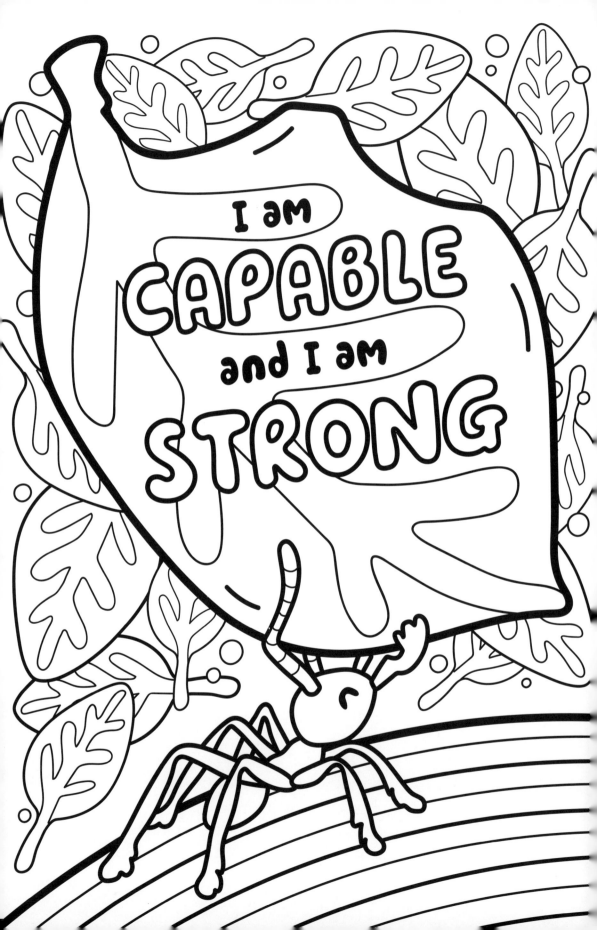

Useful distractions

It can be really hard to ignore those anxious thoughts and feelings when they arise. Here are some suggestions of distractions to help you cope with the anxiety.

- Watch something that makes you laugh
- Call a friend
- Do some exercise that you love
- Research a topic that fascinates you
- Start a DIY or craft project
- Start a blog or write in your journal
- Recite the lyrics to your favourite song out loud
- Do something productive – clean your kitchen or iron your clothes
- Care for your pets, houseplants or home
- Get stuck into a lengthy boxset you've been meaning to watch

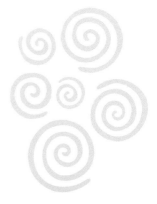

Distractions that help me

You might already have your own ideas for distraction techniques that help you. Write down some ideas that you could try if you need to take your mind off things.

1. ....
   ....

2. ....
   ....

3. ....
   ....

4. ....
   ....

5. ....
   ....

6. ....
   ....

7. ....
   ....

8. ....
   ....

9. ....
   ....

10. ....
    ....

How are you feeling today? Draw or write it out!

My support network

It's important to reach out for help when we are struggling, whether that be friends, family, mental health professionals or charities, for example. Have a think about who is in your network and who you can reach out to when you need support.

Friends:

....

....

....

....

....

....

....

Family:

....

....

....

....

....

....

Professionals:

....

....

....

....

....

....

....

Other:

....

....

....

....

....

....

....

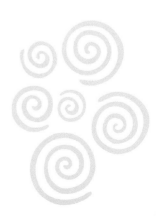

What is important to me?

When we are struggling with our mental health it can be really difficult to remember what is important to us. Try and make a list of things that are important to you.

1. ....

   ....

2. ....

   ....

3. ....

   ....

4. ....

   ....

5. ....

   ....

6. ....

   ....

7. ....

   ....

8. ....

   ....

9. ....

   ....

10. ....

What are my values?

Our values guide the way we behave, both towards others and towards ourselves. It can be useful to identify our values as this can help us to establish changes we want to make, so we can align our actions closer to the things that are important to us. Here is a list of values that you might connect with. It might help to highlight some, but there is also space to record your own that don't feature here.

Achievement	Health	Order
Adventure	Hope	Peace
Beauty	Independence	Productivity
Bravery	Individuality	Quality
Community	Intelligence	Recreation
Compassion	Joy	Reflection
Connection	Justice	Security
Dedication	Kindness	Spirituality
Discovery	Knowledge	Success
Empowerment	Learning	Teamwork
Equality	Love	Tolerance
Family	Morality	Truthfulness
Freedom	Motivation	Unity
Fun	Nourishment	Wealth
Generosity	Nurture	....
Growth	Optimism	....
....	....	....
....	....	....
....	....	....
....	....	....
....	....	....
....	....	....
....	....	....

What changes can I make that will bring me closer to living a life aligned with my values?

Are there any moves you can make to move closer to your values, such as your relationships, career, education or hobbies?

....

....

....

....

....

....

....

....

....

....

....

....

....

....

....

....

....

Brain dump

How are you feeling right now? Sometimes getting our thoughts out onto the page can help us to process and make sense of them.

....

....

....

....

....

....

....

....

....

....

....

....

....

....

....

....

....

....

....

....

Fight, flight, freeze

The fight, flight, freeze response is an innate reaction to feelings of anxiety that has been around since we were cavepeople. It is our body's physiological response to high levels of anxiety and is designed to keep us safe in dangerous situations.

When we experience anxiety, there are a number of different ways our body reacts. The hormones cortisol and adrenaline are released, which aim to make us more alert, improve our reaction times and make us stronger and faster. This allows us to fight the threat, run away from it, or play dead if we feel we are unable to escape or win in a physical altercation.

Fight, flight, freeze is not something we consciously do or can control; it is our body's way of protecting us when we feel in danger and is the cause of many of the physical symptoms we feel when we experience anxiety.

Your body wants to keep you safe and free from harm, so it reacts swiftly and strongly to feelings of fear and anxiety. If you live with panic attacks, frequent anxiety or an anxiety disorder, you will probably be somewhat in tune with your body's reaction to danger.

Fight

Fight refers to the option that would be to confront the threat head on and fight it.

Flight

Flight refers to running away or fleeing from the danger if possible.

Freeze

If we feel otherwise unable to escape the danger, or it doesn't seem as though we would win a physical altercation, we might opt to play dead. This would be referred to as freeze.

The fight, flight, freeze response is an automatic one, and you won't consciously weigh up your options, but you might become familiar with this response and experience it at times when you feel high levels of anxiety.

Now that we no longer face as many natural threats, the fight, flight, freeze response can be triggered by situations when it isn't necessarily appropriate or helpful, like a social situation, journey or event at work that doesn't require any of these three natural responses. Regardless of whether they are appropriate to what's happening around you, your body's reactions to anxiety are natural and unconscious and you shouldn't blame yourself for experiencing them.

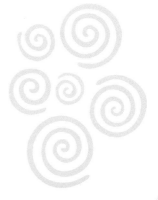

How our body reacts to anxiety

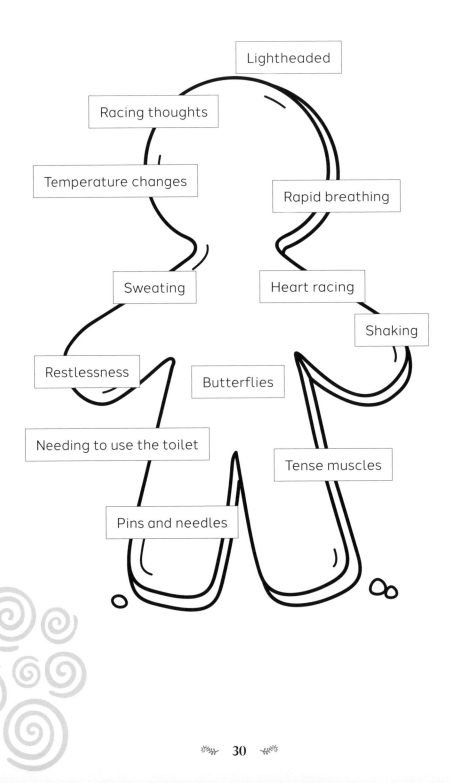

Lightheaded

Racing thoughts

Temperature changes

Rapid breathing

Sweating

Heart racing

Shaking

Restlessness

Butterflies

Needing to use the toilet

Tense muscles

Pins and needles

Signs I am feeling anxious

Everybody's experience of anxiety varies; you might feel it in different parts of your body to somebody else, for example, or behave in a different way. What are some signs that you might be feeling anxious? What do you, and the people around you, need to look out for?

....

....

....

....

....

....

....

....

....

....

....

....

....

....

....

....

....

....

What can I do to help myself when I am feeling anxious?

How can other people help me when I am feeling anxious?

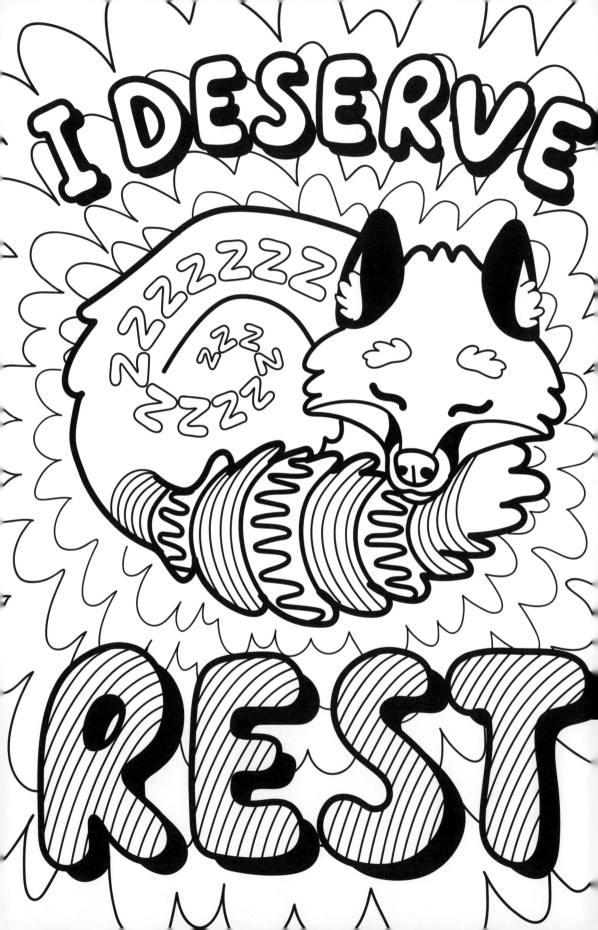

Anxiety hot cross buns

Our thoughts, feelings and behaviours all connect to one another. The way we behave can affect how we think and feel, and trying to change our thinking can impact what we do and what emotions we are experiencing. A 'hot cross bun' is a cognitive behavioural therapy-based exercise that helps us to understand ways we can and do respond in different situations, and what we could do differently next time. There is space to write down your thoughts, emotions, behaviours and physical feelings in each of the boxes. What is a situation you experience that causes you to have symptoms of anxiety?

Anxiety situation/trigger:

....

....

....

Thoughts

Physical sensations

Emotions

Behaviours

Challenging our thoughts and trying to alter the way we behave in response to difficult emotions can result in improvements to how we feel. What are some alternative thoughts and behaviours you could do in the situation you've chosen, and how might that impact your emotions?

What could I do differently in this situation?

....

....

....

Thoughts

Physical sensations

Emotions

Behaviours

Things I hate about my anxiety

⁂⁂⁂⁂⁂⁂⁂⁂⁂⁂⁂⁂⁂

It can sometimes feel difficult to want to overcome our anxiety as it can help us to feel safe, but it is through challenging it that we change it. What are some things you dislike about your anxiety that motivate you to want to make changes?

1. ....

....

2. ....

....

3. ....

....

4. ....

....

5. ....

....

6. ....

....

7. ....

....

8. ....

....

9. ....

....

10. ....

What does my anxiety currently stop me from doing?

1. ....
....
2. ....
....
3. ....
....
4. ....
....
5. ....
....
6. ....
....
7. ....
....
8. ....
....
9. ....
....
10. ....

Anxiety scale

It can be helpful when we come to thinking about different ways to face our anxiety later on, to have a scale of what different levels of anxiousness feel like to you. Starting from 1 (least anxiety) and working up to 10 (most anxiety), write down what each of those levels feels and looks like to you, and how you would know the difference between each number.

1. ....

....

....

....

2. ....

....

....

....

3. ....

....

....

....

4. ....

....

....

....

5. ....
....
....
....

6. ....
....
....
....

7. ....
....
....
....

8. ....
....
....
....

9. ....
....
....
....

10. ....
....
....
....

Coping with panic attacks

Not everybody who has difficulties with anxiety will experience panic attacks, but some people do. Symptoms of a panic attack include rapid heart rate, hyperventilation, nausea, a feeling of dread or terror, chest pain, sweating and a fear of dying. Not all of these symptoms need to be experienced simultaneously during a panic attack. They can last anywhere from five minutes to half an hour, and they can feel incredibly scary.

If you are experiencing a panic attack, the following strategies can be helpful in reducing the intensity and length of time:

✼ Concentrate on taking deep, slow breaths

✼ Try to notice what is going on around you, such as counting everything blue you can see, or how many different sounds you can hear

✼ Focus on the sensation of your feet on the floor to ground yourself

✼ Ask somebody to sit with you until it passes

✼ Remember that no matter how scary a panic attack feels, they are not dangerous and cannot hurt you

✼ Be kind to yourself once it passes – panic attacks are exhausting for your brain and your body

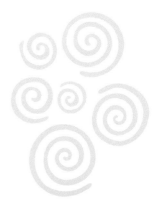

Pros and cons of change

Sometimes, you might feel that you don't want to make changes – this is a normal feeling, and lots of people will experience it. It can be helpful to weigh up the pros and cons of making recovery-focused decisions, as this can help you to reflect on the benefits of challenging your anxiety.

What are the pros of recovering?

....
....
....
....
....
....
....
....

What are the cons of recovering?

....
....
....
....
....
....
....

What are the pros of not recovering?

....

....

....

....

....

....

....

....

What are the cons of not recovering?

....

....

....

....

....

....

....

....

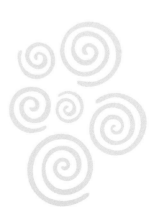

Therapeutic crafting – crochet

Crochet is a great creative activity for anxious people because it's engaging enough to help provide distraction, while still being a gentle activity that won't leave you feeling overwhelmed or overstimulated. There are so many wonderful tutorials and patterns out there, and it's a fairly inexpensive hobby to get started – all you need is some yarn and a crochet hook! I learned to crochet by following Bella Coco's tutorials on YouTube – her 'granny square for beginners' video is a great place to start.

Once you've learned the basics, you'll be able to work on your projects while watching your favourite TV shows or listening to interesting podcasts – meaning that you can layer comforting hobbies to create some truly relaxing self-care days. You can channel a lot of nervous energy into the repetitive movements (plus it keeps your hands busy!) so it really is especially helpful for anxious people who struggle with skin picking or hair pulling.

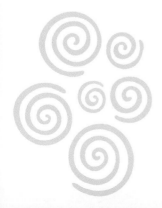

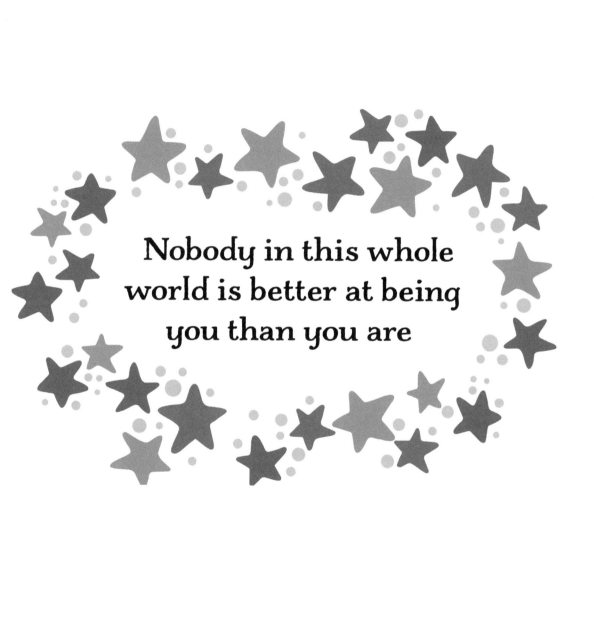

Nobody in this whole
world is better at being
you than you are

How are you feeling today? Draw or write it out!

Letter writing

It can feel really overwhelming to be very anxious and fearful. What would you like to say to yourself next time you're struggling with feelings of anxiety?

....

....

....

....

....

....

....

....

....

....

....

....

....

....

....

....

....

....

....

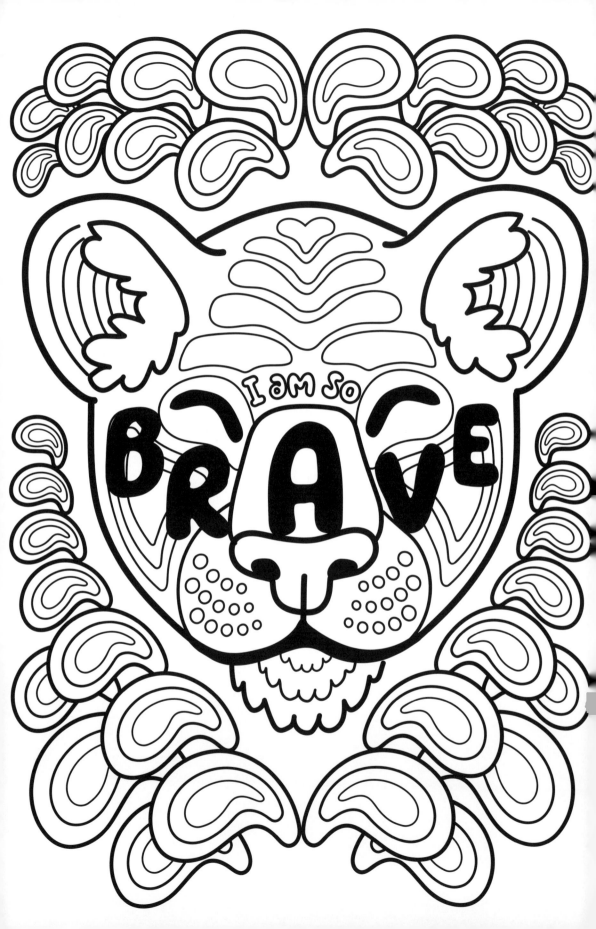

Calming activities

What do you do that helps you to feel calm and reduce your levels of anxiety? Is there anything you can try that you haven't already?

....

....

....

....

....

....

....

....

....

....

....

....

....

....

....

....

....

....

....

....

Brain dump

How are you feeling right now? Sometimes getting our thoughts out onto the page can help us to process and make sense of them.

....

....

....

....

....

....

....

....

....

....

....

....

....

....

....

....

....

....

....

Nourishing ourselves

Learning to create your favourite meals, snacks or treats from scratch is a freeing experience. It's a fantastic way to invest in yourself and your health, show yourself some love and get creative. Plus you get the bonus of eating what you make and potentially saving yourself some money along the way.

One of the great things about cooking is that you can really choose how adventurous you are feeling. From following a simple recipe to experimenting with a variety of exotic ingredients to booking yourself into a local class – cooking is a fantastic creative pursuit that will allow you to nourish yourself and those you love. Creative *and* practical.

Stuck for ideas? Here are some delicious recipes to inspire you and tickle your tastebuds!

Savoury:

- ❧ Barbecued sweetcorn ribs with plantain hummus: www.bbc.co.uk/food/recipes/barbecued_sweetcorn_ribs_81012

- ❧ Easy dairy-free creamy tomato pasta: www.itsmorefuninyour30s.wordpress.com/2023/03/05/recipe-easy-dairy-free-creamy-tomato-pasta

- ❧ Mushroom and broccoli stir fry: www.bbc.co.uk/food/recipes/mushroom_and_broccoli_33092

- ❧ Steph's chickpea curry with spinach and rice: www.pinchofyum.com/chickpea-curry

Sweet:

- ❧ Almond flour brownies: www.hummingbirdhigh.com/2021/01/small-batch-almond-flour-brownies.html

- ❧ Easy overnight oats: www.feelgoodfoodie.net/recipe/overnight-oats

❀ Snickerdoodle cookies: www.loveandlemons.com/snickerdoodle-recipe

Keep an eye out for DIY food kits from your favourite restaurants too as many offer them, and it means that you can have food you already know you love at home and can learn from chefs that you trust!

What does my anxiety look like?

Try drawing it below.

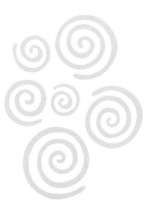

What is worry?

Worry and anxiety are often used as interchangeable terms, but they do in fact have slightly different meanings. Whilst anxiety is the emotion we experience and that causes the physical response in our body, worry is the thought process that occurs in our minds. It usually consists of ruminating on future events and what the potential negative outcomes of these will be.

Worry is more likely to occur when the situation is new, or the outcomes aren't clear or feel unpredictable. Worry is a common cognitive process and one everybody will experience from time to time, but it can become problematic if it is stopping you from living the life you want to live. This might be because it feels disproportionate, excessive or frequent, and it is getting in the way of day-to-day activities.

Worry jar

Sometimes, the number of different worries we have can feel over-whelming. Try getting yourself a jar, box or envelope. Each time you experience a worry, write it down and put it away. The act of filing away a worry can be helpful in allowing us to separate it from ourselves and is symbolic of letting it go. Revisiting these at a later date can also be a useful reminder that often our worries, however scary they feel at the time, are not proportionate, and the events we fear often pass uneventfully.

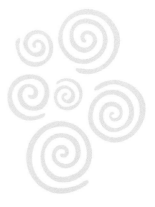

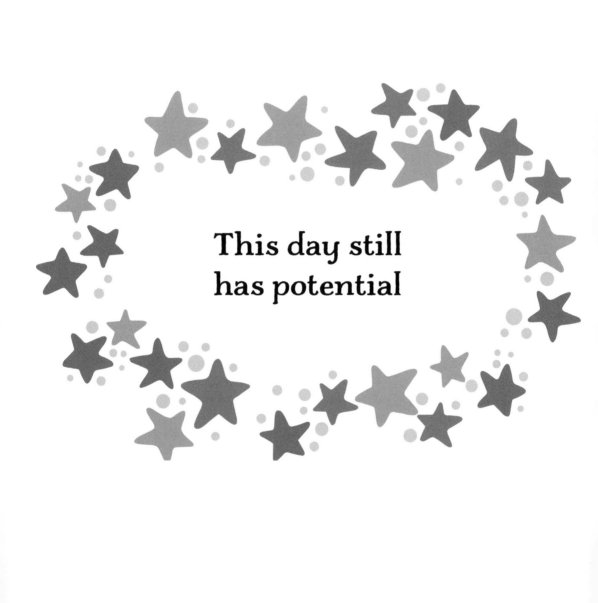

This day still
has potential

Worry chaining

People who experience high levels of anxiety often do something called worry chaining. Most worry starts with the question 'what if?', and this can cause a chain or spiral of worry until we are focusing on the worst-case scenario or have a series of unpredictable options that we feel anxious about. An example of this might be preparing to take an exam and going through the following thought process.

- What if I haven't studied enough?
- What if I don't do well in the exam?
- What if I get into trouble?
- What if I fail my course?
- What if I can't get the job I want?
- What if I can't get a job at all?
- What if I can't make any money?
- What if I can't afford my house?

Think of a situation in which you notice yourself worry chaining. Write it down here:

....

....

Now add to it with 'what if's':

What if... ....

What if... ....

What if... ....

What if... ....

What if... ....

Challenging worry

There are questions we can ask ourselves to try to challenge those worry thoughts as they arise. Try and use the format below to challenge a worry you experience.

What is the worry?

....

....

What evidence do I have that the worry will come true?

....

....

What evidence do I have that the worry won't come true?

....

....

What is the most likely outcome?

....

....

If my worry does come true, how can I cope?

....

....

If my worry does come true, will it still matter a week, a month or a year from now?

....

....

Is worry useful?

One reason people might find the idea of challenging their worry thoughts difficult, and feel reluctant to do this, is that they believe there are some benefits to worry and anxiety. These can include:

- ❀ Worrying helps me to problem solve
- ❀ Worrying helps motivate me to do things
- ❀ Worrying stops bad things from happening
- ❀ Worrying helps me perform better
- ❀ Worrying shows I care about things
- ❀ Worrying is a positive personality trait
- ❀ Worry protects me from negative emotions

These thoughts can often be difficult to overcome, and we may be able to gather evidence that convinces us they are true. However, there are often many more negatives to worry than positives. Try asking yourself some of the following questions:

- ❀ Do I get better results compared to people who worry less than I do?
- ❀ Does my worry interfere with my relationships?
- ❀ Can I think of times I have had positive outcomes when I haven't worried?
- ❀ Have there been any times that my worry hasn't prevented negative outcomes?
- ❀ Has worry ever had a negative impact on my school or work performance?
- ❀ Do I spend a lot of time and energy worrying?
- ❀ Do I know people who are successful who don't worry as much as I do?
- ❀ Does worry ever cause me to feel tired and fatigued?
- ❀ Does worry ever solve my problems?
- ❀ Am I able to stop myself worrying?
- ❀ Does worrying ever cost me anything?

Collage making

Making a collage is such a simple and beginner-friendly creative art form that you can get stuck into. A collage can be made up of magazine cuttings, printed pictures, paintings, poems, stickers, photographs, fabrics, wood and pretty much any other material you can get your hands on. The key is to make the process as enjoyable and flexible as you can, while following your intuition.

Allow yourself to be drawn to the images or items that attract you and then experiment with layers, texture and composition until you've arranged your items in a way that feels pleasing to you. When you really lose yourself in the process, you'll find that you can make beautiful and inspiring things that come together at your own pace. It can be a really sensory process.

If you already enjoy making mood boards, vision boards or even Pinterest boards, then you'll really enjoy this activity.

Here are some collage ideas you might enjoy putting together if you're in need of inspiration:

❀ A collage that represents a time or place that you felt completely at ease – it could include natural materials you collected, photographs, train tickets and maps!

❀ A visual collage that shows off your favourite band, book or movie – you could use promotional materials, press cuttings, printed photographs, quotes or lyrics

❀ An ode to your favourite painter or artist – search for interviews with the artist, biographical information on their life, magazine pages that feature their work and try to recreate some of their signature techniques yourself

❀ Make a giant rainbow, or create something entirely monochrome in your favourite colour – group items together by colour rather than theme and arrange them in a pleasing way on a canvas, card or piece of wood

✤ Thousands of dogs. Or cats. Or otters. Choose your favourite animal and just find as many cute pictures of them as you can. I bet this one will make you super happy to do!

Don't stop there – inspiration can be found anywhere, and virtually anything can be turned into a collage. Your favourite interests, your heritage, your family, different periods of history, plants you think are beautiful, food you've enjoyed, different aesthetic themes and even something as simple as a certain number – these can all make beautiful and intricate collages that will keep you busy for hours.

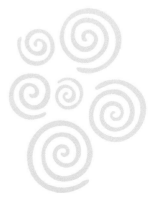

Current vs hypothetical worries

Worry generally falls into two categories: current problems and hypothetical situations.

Current problems are focused on concerns that are happening in the here and now. This might include worrying about passing an assignment you're doing, or being off sick from work and worrying about money.

Hypothetical worries involve focusing on situations that do not yet exist, and in many cases never will. For example, this may include worrying about crashing your car on the way to work, or fearing a friend may become sick.

As current worries involve real and present situations, that often means there are things we are able to do to problem solve them. This might look like setting yourself time aside every day to focus on your assignment, or budgeting to account for reduced sick pay.

Hypothetical worries can present more of a challenge, as we cannot problem solve situations that do not exist.

The way we challenge each of these types of worry is different. To cope with current worries, we need to use problem-solving skills, whereas hypothetical worries require us to face our fears and complete exposure exercises. We will address both of these strategies later on in this book.

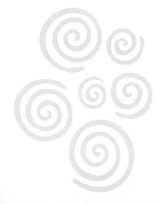

My worries

What are some of your main worries? Do you think they are current problems or hypothetical situations?

Worry	Current or hypothetical?
. . . .	. . . .
. . . .	. . . .
. . . .	. . . .
. . . .	. . . .
. . . .	. . . .
. . . .	. . . .
. . . .	. . . .
. . . .	. . . .
. . . .	. . . .
. . . .	. . . .
. . . .	. . . .
. . . .	. . . .
. . . .	. . . .
. . . .	. . . .
. . . .	. . . .
. . . .	. . . .
. . . .	. . . .
. . . .	. . . .
. . . .	. . . .

Worry tree

Worry trees can help us identify whether a problem is a current or hypothetical worry, and then figure out a plan of what we can do about it. Try using the below decision tree to help you make a plan for your worry.

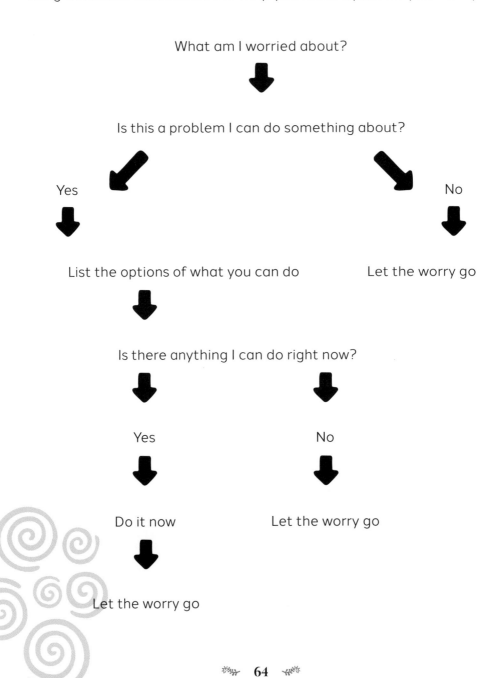

What am I worried about?

Is this a problem I can do something about?

Yes

No

List the options of what you can do

Let the worry go

Is there anything I can do right now?

Yes

No

Do it now

Let the worry go

Let the worry go

Circle of control

It can help reduce our anxiety if we pay attention to things we can control, vs things we can't. For example, we can control our own behaviour, but we can't control other people's responses to our behaviour. Try writing down things you are in control of inside the inner circle, things you have some control over in the middle circle, and the things you are not in control in the outer circle.

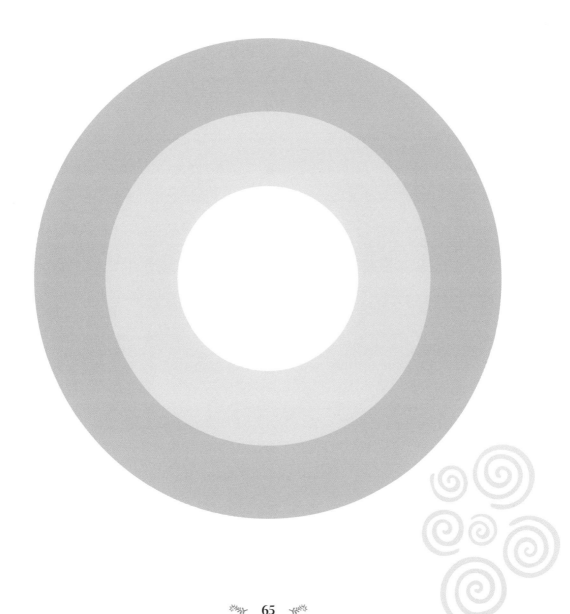

How are you feeling today? Draw or write it out!

Coping statements

Coping statements are phrases we can say to ourselves when we are feeling like things are getting overwhelming. Try using some of these next time things are feeling difficult.

1. It's good to acknowledge my thoughts and feelings. This is my body responding to those thoughts and feelings.

2. I recognize these symptoms. I have experienced them before.

3. I am safe, and I know how to keep myself safe.

4. It is okay that I am struggling right now, and it is okay for me to just focus on getting through this.

5. I have survived all of my bad days, and I will survive today.

6. I am only scared of the future because I know that I matter and my future matters.

7. Not all of my thoughts are helpful or true.

8. I am creative, and I am capable of imagining scary scenarios, but this does not mean that they will come true.

9. I won't feel like this forever.

10. The people who matter will not judge me for not being okay.

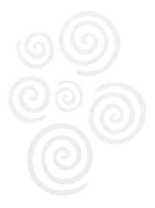

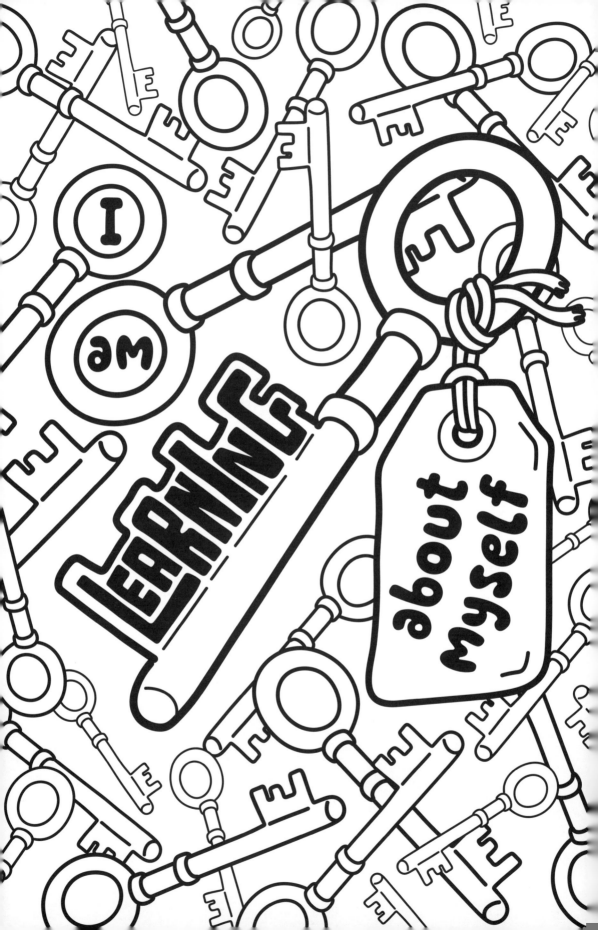

I am LEARNING about myself

Worry time

Worry time is the act of setting aside some time where you allow yourself to worry, so that it doesn't become the focus of your day. It can take some practice but can be an effective strategy at managing worry so that it doesn't become overwhelming.

Try setting aside 15–30 minutes a day, preferably at a regular time, in a place that feels neutral. Allow yourself to think about your worries in this time, but arrange an activity following it so that you are able to distract yourself from those thoughts.

Over the course of the day, each time you notice a worry, write it down and then divert your attention away from it. During worry time, you can come back to the notes you have made.

During worry time, you can spend time establishing whether your worries are current or hypothetical and make plans to resolve them.

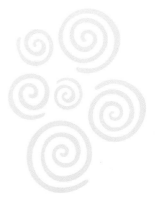

Safety behaviours

Safety behaviours are things we do to help lower our anxiety in chal-lenging situations. This might include things like excessive checking, reassurance seeking, not doing things alone or even avoiding things altogether. Everyone's safety behaviours are individual to them. The problem with these behaviours is that although they make us less anx-ious in the short term, in the long run they keep us stuck. For example, if we only ever attend social events with another person, we don't get to find out if we would cope alone.

Have a think and identify some of your safety behaviours. For each one, think about how you can start to challenge it.

Safety behaviour:

....

....

How can I challenge this?

....

....

Safety behaviour:

....

....

How can I challenge this?

....

....

Safety behaviour:

....

....

How can I challenge this?

....

....

Safety behaviour:

....

....

How can I challenge this?

....

....

Safety behaviour:

....

....

How can I challenge this?

....

....

Safety behaviour:

....

....

How can I challenge this?

....

....

Creative construction

Construction is a very satisfying creative activity because it allows you to make something tangible. If you're looking for a hobby that will allow you to learn and explore a range of skills and mediums, look no further than construction.

You can practise construction using some basic wooden blocks, craft and paint a detailed model aeroplane from a kit or even create an elaborate miniature landscape.

Whichever form of construction appeals to you the most, it is guaranteed to be a very involved process that requires focus and dedication.

If you're not sure what you'd like to create, opt for a simple and reusable interlocking building block (like Lego®) so that you can experiment with the kind of structures and shapes that are enjoyable to you. The amount of focus this activity requires will help you keep your thoughts on the task at hand.

Things I like about myself

Low self-esteem is often something that occurs alongside mental health difficulties. Try to think of some qualities you like about yourself that you can reflect on in future.

1. ....
....

2. ....
....

3. ....
....

4. ....
....

5. ....
....

6. ....
....

7. ....
....

8. ....
....

9. ....
....

10. ....
....

Things other people like about me

It can also be helpful to reflect on things other people value in us, as they may be different to our own. Ask the people around you what they like about you and write them below – some of the answers might surprise you.

1. ....
....

2. ....
....

3. ....
....

4. ....
....

5. ....
....

6. ....
....

7. ....
....

8. ....
....

9. ....
....

10. ....
....

Self-care activities

It can feel difficult to look after ourselves when we are struggling with our mental health. One of the best ways to challenge this is to start being kind to ourselves. What self-care activities can you try?

1. ....

    ....

2. ....

    ....

3. ....

    ....

4. ....

    ....

5. ....

    ....

6. ....

    ....

7. ....

    ....

8. ....

    ....

9. ....

    ....

10. ....

    ....

31 days of self-care

1 Take a moment to breathe deeply and stretch your body	2 Remind yourself that you are powerful – say it out loud	3 Be as tall as you can be today. You should be proud of how far you've come
8 Spend some time in nature	9 Gently stroke your face and body – you deserve kindness	10 Wake up earlier and enjoy a slow morning
15 Treat yourself to a special meal this evening	16 Pamper yourself and spend time on your skin today	17 Unfollow social media accounts that make you feel bad
22 Listen to an interesting podcast	23 Find some quiet time to drink a nice hot drink	24 Watch the sunset or sunrise
29 Book an appointment you've been meaning to book	30 List 10 things you think you're really good at	31 Schedule some more self-care ideas in your calendar

4 Think about a place you felt content and calm – what makes that place so calming?	5 Tell a loved one what they mean to you	6 Make a special effort to go to bed on time	7 Watch an episode of your favourite comfort show
11 Complete a task you've been putting off	12 Read or listen to a chapter of a new book	13 Reach out to a friend	14 Write down three things you are grateful for
18 Make a list of achievable short-term goals	19 Rewatch your favourite movie	20 Plan and take yourself on a date	21 Declutter an area of your home that is causing you stress
25 Move your body in a way that feels fun and safe	26 Listen to your favourite song	27 Do something that brought you joy as a child	28 Write a list of people who inspire you

Miracle question

If you woke up tomorrow and your anxiety was completely gone, what would your day look like?

....

....

....

....

....

....

....

....

....

....

....

....

....

....

....

....

....

....

....

Happy memories

Can you think of any times you have managed to challenge your anxiety that have worked out positively? What memories have you created in doing this?

....

....

....

....

....

....

....

....

....

....

....

....

....

....

....

....

....

....

....

....

Progressive muscle relaxation

Progressive muscle relaxation is a strategy that can be used to reduce feelings of stress and anxiety. It is a simple exercise to follow, and it can be helpful to set time aside every day to practise so that when it is needed, you can remember what to do. Try following these instructions, laying down on a flat surface, working from your toes to your head:

Feet: Curl up your toes then release them, one foot at a time

Calves: Point and flex your feet, one leg at a time

Knees: Lock your knees then release them, one knee at a time

Thighs: Squeeze your thighs together tightly, then release them

Stomach: Suck in your stomach, then let it go

Back: Squeeze your shoulder blades together, then release them

Hands: Clench your fists then stretch out your fingers, one hand at a time

Elbows: Lock your elbows, then release them, one arm at a time

Shoulders: Hunch your shoulders, then let them relax

Neck: Slowly move your head as though you are looking up to the sky, then down towards your chest

Jaw: Clench your jaw, then release it

Face: Scrunch up your face, then relax it

You should hold each tension for 10 seconds, then allow your body to relax for 20 seconds. While relaxing your body, notice the changes you can feel in the area of your body you have been tensing. Breathe deeply and move on to the next body part. As you release the tension, try to imagine your anxiety leaving that part of your body.

How are you feeling today? Draw or write it out!

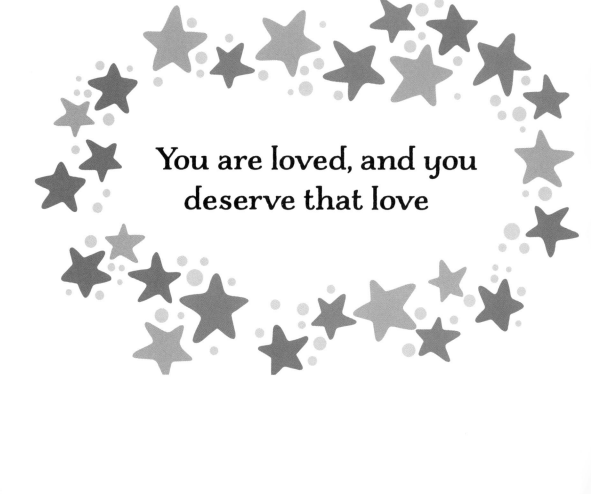

You are loved, and you deserve that love

Current coping strategies

It's likely that over time you will have picked up some coping strategies for when things get difficult. However, it's important to remember that these might not always be healthy or beneficial to us in the long term, even though they might help us in the short term. Hopefully, you will also have some strategies that are helpful for you both now and in the future. Have a think through the coping strategies you currently use when you are anxious, and whether these are helpful for both present and future you.

Coping strategy:

....
....
....

Short-term pros:

....
....
....

Short-term cons:

....
....
....

Long-term pros:

....
....
....

Long-term cons:

....
....
....

Coping strategy:

....
....
....

Short-term pros:

....
....
....

Short-term cons:

....
....
....

Long-term pros:

. . . .

. . . .

. . . .

Long-term cons:

. . . .

. . . .

. . . .

Coping strategy:

. . . .

. . . .

. . . .

Short-term pros:

. . . .

. . . .

. . . .

Short-term cons:

. . . .

. . . .

. . . .

Long-term pros:

. . . .

. . . .

. . . .

Long-term cons:

. . . .

. . . .

. . . .

New coping strategies

Are there any coping strategies that you haven't tried yet, that you think might be helpful? List them below, and revisit this page next time you feel you need it.

1. ....
   ....

2. ....
   ....

3. ....
   ....

4. ....
   ....

5. ....
   ....

6. ....
   ....

7. ....
   ....

8. ....
   ....

9. ....
   ....

10. ....
    ....

Positive self-talk

Positive self-talk can be really challenging to do when we feel anxious and worried. It involves listening to and noticing our thoughts, and identifying statements that can challenge them.

Some positive self-talk statements include:

- I can do this

- I have been anxious before and got through it

- Anxiety can't hurt me

- I have coped with difficult situations before

- I am brave

- It's okay if things aren't perfect

- I've done this once, so I can do it again

- I can only try my best

Can you think of any more?

....

....

....

....

....

....

....

....

....

....

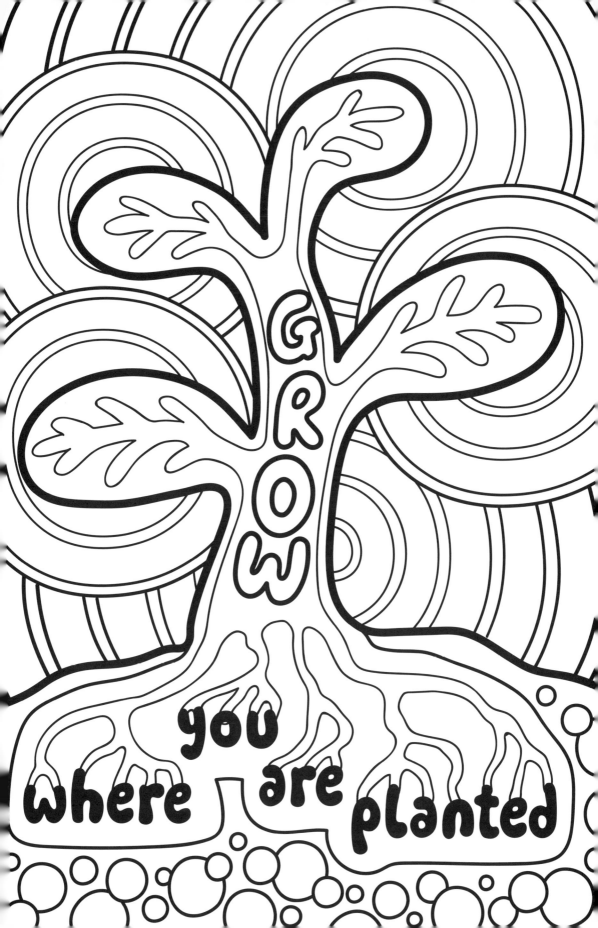

54321 grounding technique

Anxiety and distress can feel completely overwhelming sometimes. If you find yourself feeling like this, this technique can be very effective at bringing you back into the here and now by helping you to connect to your senses. There are five steps to follow.

1. Look around you and notice **five things you can see**. This could be a painting, a plant or a person, for example. Pay attention to what each of these things look like: their shapes, colours and sizes.

2. Focus on **four things you can feel**. This could be the wind, your clothes against your skin, the floor underneath your feet. Notice the different textures and sensations.

3. Name **three things you can hear**. Maybe there are birds chirping outside, or cars passing in the street. Perhaps you can hear a TV show in the background. Focus on the different tones and volumes.

4. Notice **two things you can smell**. Have you used a nice fabric softener on your clothes, or are you wearing your favourite perfume? Maybe you are outdoors and can smell plants and flowers.

5. Think about one **thing you can taste**. Perhaps you have chewing gum or a cup of tea nearby. If you can't taste anything, try to imagine what one of your favourite things tastes like.

Calming painting

You don't have to be a talented artist to be able to paint for your anxiety. Painting can be an intuitive and emotional process that will allow you to experiment with shapes, colours and techniques in order to let go of some of the thoughts and feelings that are troubling you.

Through painting, it is often possible to visualize or depict different feelings that we are experiencing, and many artists have reported it as being a safe way to express and explore emotions.

You can choose to use the painting process to influence your mood directly by using soothing tones and colours to create calming shapes and imagery that help you unwind.

Or you might choose to let some of the more anxious emotions out onto the canvas as a therapeutic and visual way of letting them go. Experiment and find out what works for you!

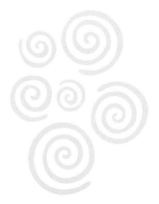

The power of music

Music can be an amazing tool for our wellbeing, and there are so many inspiring songs and artists out there. The type of music we listen to can have a big impact on our mood, and it would be helpful to think about what songs might help you when you need a bit of motivation to challenge yourself, as well as when you feel you need some calm and peace.

My motivational playlist:

....

....

....

....

....

....

....

....

My calming playlist:

....

....

....

....

....

....

....

....

Coping with uncertainty

One of the reasons people with anxiety struggle so much with worrying about future events is that often situations can feel unpredictable, and the outcomes are not set in stone. This leads to people trying to increase the certainty of the outcome by doing things like reassurance seeking, excessive planning or avoidance of situations altogether. Rather than trying to increase the certainty of particular outcomes, what we need to be focusing on is increasing our tolerance to things being uncertain.

There are two main reasons that uncertainty feels threatening to people who struggle with anxiety. The first of these is the belief that uncertain events will have negative outcomes. The second is that they believe that they have an inability to cope with negative outcomes if they do occur.

Intolerance of uncertainty can manifest in two ways – we call these 'approach' or 'avoidance' strategies.

Approach strategies include:

❄ Taking control of situations and not allowing others to contribute
❄ Doing lots of research before completing a task
❄ Seeking reassurance from others
❄ Excessively checking or repeating things to make sure they are correct

Avoidance strategies include:

❄ Not committing fully to things
❄ Procrastinating
❄ Finding reasons not to do things, whether real or imaginary
❄ Difficulty making decisions

Uncertainty is part of life, and no matter what measures we take, we cannot make every outcome in life certain. It can help to think about the benefits of uncertainty. Would life be boring without it? Have you ever experienced a positive outcome from something you were uncertain about? Try answering the following questions to have a think about your own attitudes towards uncertainty.

What advantages are there to being certain about things?

....

....

....

Are there any advantages to uncertainty?

....

....

....

Are there any disadvantages to always being certain?

....

....

....

Are there any uncertainties in your life
that you are able to cope with?

....

....

....

The way we can build up our tolerance to feeling uncertain is by first identifying what we do to try to reduce our anxiety and increase certainty (these are our safety behaviours). Next, we need to expose ourselves to uncertain situations, which increases our tolerance to anxiety and teaches us that we are able to cope with unpredictability, regardless of the outcome. We do this by creating a hierarchy of situations to challenge ourselves with, which we will come to later on in this book.

My skills and strengths

Everybody has their own individual strengths that we can draw upon when things feel difficult. What are some of yours? If you feel stuck, it can help to ask the people around you their thoughts.

1. ....
....

2. ....
....

3. ....
....

4. ....
....

5. ....
....

6. ....
....

7. ....
....

8. ....
....

9. ....
....

10. ....
....

Brain dump

How are you feeling right now? Sometimes getting our thoughts out onto the page can help us to process and make sense of them.

....

....

....

....

....

....

....

....

....

....

....

....

....

....

....

....

....

....

....

....

Problem solving

Often, the experience of a fear of uncertainty is because people with anxiety are not confident in their ability to be able to problem solve. Sometimes it can help to break down different solutions to a problem, as this can then lead to us being able to identify the pros and cons of each outcome in order to come to a decision. Try using this table to explore a worry you currently have.

What is the worry?		
What is a potential solution?	**What are the benefits to this?**	**What are the cons of this?**
What solution have I chosen and why?		

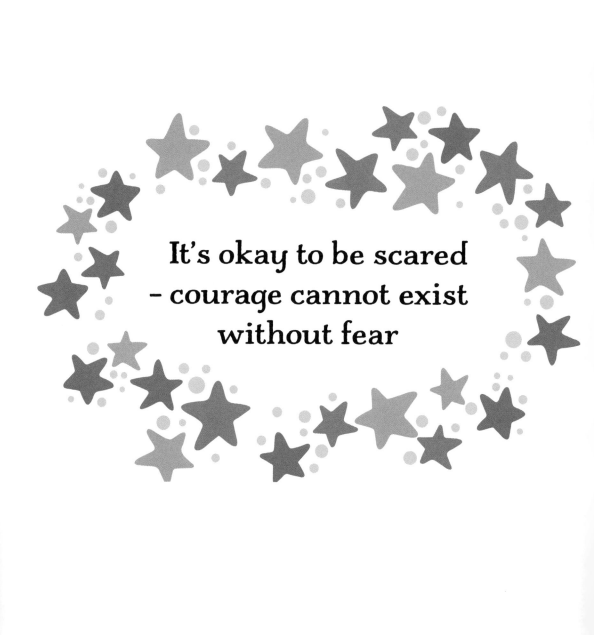

It's okay to be scared
- courage cannot exist
without fear

Square breathing technique

Square breathing has been shown to be helpful when trying to relax and feel calm, and it is an exercise that can be used wherever you are. Find a window, a wall, a painting or any other square shape you can see to focus on. If you can't see one, you can use your index finger to trace one in front of you.

Slowly trace your eyes across the top of the square in front of you, breathing in for a count of four. As you scan down the right side of the square, hold your breath for a count of four. Breathe out for a count of four as you trace the bottom of the square, then hold for a count of four as you scan up the left-hand side. Repeat this as many times as necessary, breathing in a slow and controlled way.

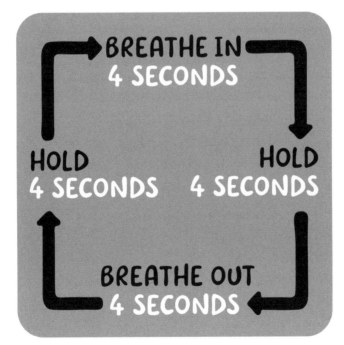

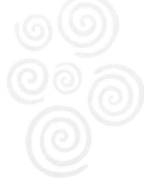

Unhelpful thinking traps

Most of us have thinking habits we have developed over our lives that can sometimes get in the way when we are feeling distressing and difficult emotions. These are some of the most common ones that people experience.

Mind reading:

Assuming we know what other people are thinking.

Example: 'They all think I am stupid.'

Ask yourself: Am I making assumptions about what they are thinking?

Prediction:

Thinking we know what's going to happen in the future.

Example: 'I am going to fail that assignment.'

Ask yourself: How likely is it that this is going to happen?

Comparing and despairing:

Only seeing the positives in others then comparing ourselves against them negatively.

Example: 'I am rubbish at drawing compared to them.'

Ask yourself: Am I focusing on others rather than myself?

Mental filter:

Only noticing what we want to notice and filtering out everything else that doesn't fit that narrative, like sieving out all the positives and only letting the negatives through.

Example: Only noticing things we consider to be our failures and ignoring any successes.

Ask yourself: Am I only noticing the bad things?

Mountains and molehills:

Exaggerating the negatives and minimizing the positives.

Example: Thinking the negatives are worse than they are and the positives are less significant than they are.

Ask yourself: What would somebody else say about this situation?

Critical self:

Putting ourselves down and blaming ourselves for things that are not our fault; also referred to as the 'internal bully'.

Example: 'The group project not going well at work is all my fault.'

Ask yourself: What role did others play in this situation?

Shoulds and musts:

Putting pressure on ourselves and having unreasonable or unrealistic expectations of what we should or shouldn't be doing.

Example: 'I should be good at this by now.'

Ask yourself: Is this an unrealistic expectation I am setting for myself?

Black and white thinking:

Thinking that things can only be right or wrong, good or bad, with nothing in between.

Example: 'If I don't do this perfectly then I have failed.'

Ask yourself: Is it possible to do everything perfectly all of the time?

Catastrophizing:

Believing or imagining only the worst possible case scenario.

Example: 'This is going to be a disaster.'

Ask yourself: What are some other possible outcomes to this situation?

Labelling:

Giving labels to others or to ourselves.

Example: 'I am an idiot.'

Ask yourself: What would somebody else say in this situation?

Emotional reasoning:

Assuming our feelings are always rational, e.g. 'I am anxious so I must be in danger.'

Example: 'I feel ashamed so I must be a bad person.'

Ask yourself: Does feeling bad mean someone is bad?

Overgeneralizing:

Noticing a pattern based on one situation or drawing wide-ranging conclusions.

Example: 'Nothing good ever happens.'

Ask yourself: What positive things have happened?

Personalization:

Taking responsibility or feeling a sense of blame for something that may not be your fault.

Example: 'It's my fault that my friendship group fell out.'

Ask yourself: Were there any other factors involved in this situation happening?

Everybody has their own individual traps – you might find some of these don't apply to you at all, and others make complete sense. It might be helpful to think about which of them feel relevant to you, and situations where you think they might arise. For example, if you find yourself feeling very anxious about things that could happen in the future, you might be 'catastrophizing' or 'predicting'. The more you start to recognize your own thinking traps, the more you can start to challenge them.

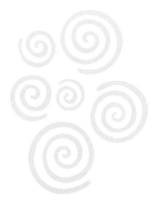

What are my unhelpful thinking styles?

When might I notice them?

....

....

....

....

....

....

....

....

....

....

....

....

....

....

....

....

....

....

....

....

How does this affect me?

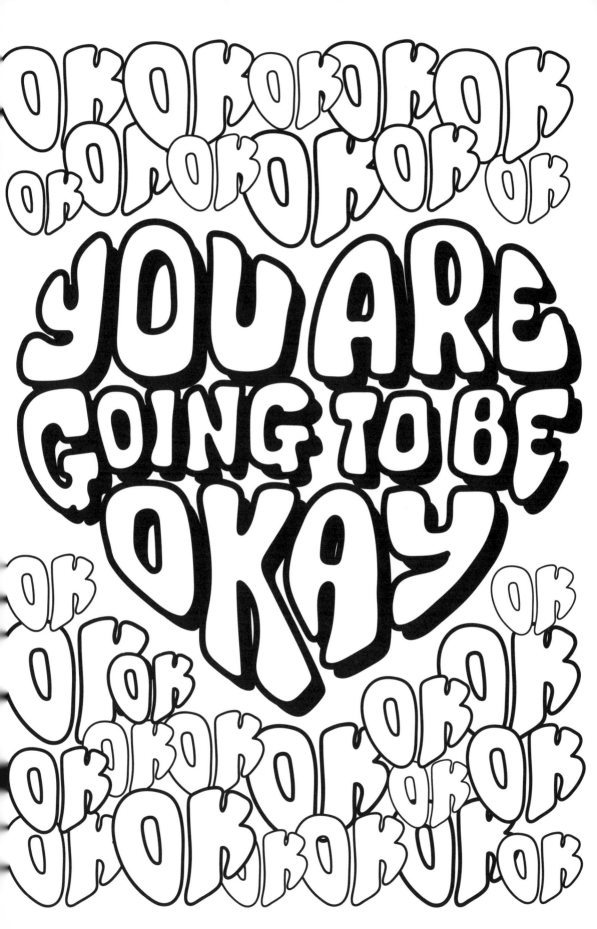

Taking on the scientist role

Part of moving forward with recovery from anxiety is conducting experiments. We can do this by creating a hierarchy of things we want to challenge, and then plan out what we are trying to achieve by doing this. On the next few pages we will start to put together a ladder of anxiety-provoking situations, before starting to put on our scientist hats and carrying out some experiments that challenge your anxiety.

On the next few pages, put together a list of situations that might be difficult for you and that raise your anxiety. It is through doing these experiments that we can build up more evidence about whether what we are worried about is likely to happen, and whether we are able to cope with difficult situations.

Some examples might be:

❀ Asking for something in a shop

❀ Calling somebody on the phone

❀ Going out without checking directions multiple times

❀ Only confirming a time and meeting place once

❀ Applying for a new job

❀ Submitting a piece of work without checking it

❀ Sending an email without looking back for mistakes

❀ Eating somewhere new without looking at the menu in advance

❀ Walking a different route to work

❀ Meeting friends without checking what other people are wearing

Everybody's experience of anxiety is unique, and you will have your own personal fears and worries, but hopefully the above suggestions will act as a prompt to help you to come up with some of your own.

Following this, we can start practising these experiments using the worksheets on the subsequent pages.

Why do we do experiments?

When we experience unknown situations, our anxiety increases. This is when we are likely to use the safety behaviours we identified earlier on. Using a safety behaviour decreases our anxiety, so we learn that this is an effective strategy for short-term management and continue using these behaviours each time we are faced with an anxiety-provoking situation.

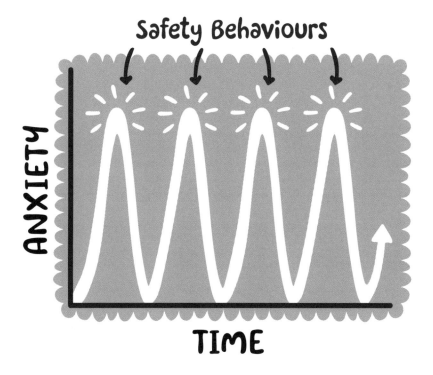

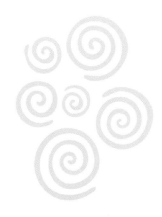

Through doing this, we never get to find out what happens if we don't use the safety behaviour, and whether our worries about negative outcomes are going to come true.

Through the act of doing behavioural experiments, we are trying to learn whether our feared outcome might not happen. Each time we practise this, our anxiety gradually starts to come down. Eventually, after lots of practice, we might notice that we feel much less anxious when in a challenging situation, and that our anxiety passes a lot quicker.

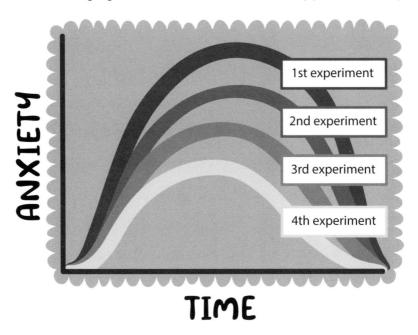

On the next few pages, we can create our hierarchy, then begin recording the outcomes of these experiments.

	Experiment	Level of anxiety (0–100%)
1.		
2.		
3.		
4.		
5.		
6.		
7.		
8.		
9.		
10.		

What am I going to do?

....

....

What am I worried is going to happen?

....

....

How anxious do I feel beforehand? (0–100%)

....

What actually happened?

....

....

Was my prediction correct?

....

....

What did I learn?

....

....

How anxious do I feel afterwards (0–100%)?

....

Do I need to repeat the experiment?

....

....

Do I need to do anything differently next time?

....

....

What am I going to do?

....

....

What am I worried is going to happen?

....

....

How anxious do I feel beforehand? (0–100%)

....

What actually happened?

....

....

Was my prediction correct?

....

....

What did I learn?

....

....

How anxious do I feel afterwards (0–100%)?

....

Do I need to repeat the experiment?

....

....

Do I need to do anything differently next time?

....

....

What am I going to do?

....

....

What am I worried is going to happen?

....

....

How anxious do I feel beforehand? (0–100%)

....

What actually happened?

....

....

Was my prediction correct?

....

....

What did I learn?

....

....

How anxious do I feel afterwards (0–100%)?

....

Do I need to repeat the experiment?

....

....

Do I need to do anything differently next time?

....

....

What am I going to do?

....

....

What am I worried is going to happen?

....

....

How anxious do I feel beforehand? (0–100%)

....

What actually happened?

....

....

Was my prediction correct?

....

....

What did I learn?

....

....

How anxious do I feel afterwards (0–100%)?

....

Do I need to repeat the experiment?

....

....

Do I need to do anything differently next time?

....

....

What am I going to do?

....

....

What am I worried is going to happen?

....

....

How anxious do I feel beforehand? (0–100%)

....

What actually happened?

....

....

Was my prediction correct?

....

....

What did I learn?

....

....

How anxious do I feel afterwards (0–100%)?

....

Do I need to repeat the experiment?

....

....

Do I need to do anything differently next time?

....

....

What am I going to do?

....

....

What am I worried is going to happen?

....

....

How anxious do I feel beforehand? (0–100%)

....

What actually happened?

....

....

Was my prediction correct?

....

....

What did I learn?

....

....

How anxious do I feel afterwards (0–100%)?

....

Do I need to repeat the experiment?

....

....

Do I need to do anything differently next time?

....

....

What am I going to do?

....

....

What am I worried is going to happen?

....

....

How anxious do I feel beforehand? (0–100%)

....

What actually happened?

....

....

Was my prediction correct?

....

....

What did I learn?

....

....

How anxious do I feel afterwards (0–100%)?

....

Do I need to repeat the experiment?

....

....

Do I need to do anything differently next time?

....

....

What am I going to do?

....

....

What am I worried is going to happen?

....

....

How anxious do I feel beforehand? (0–100%)

....

What actually happened?

....

....

Was my prediction correct?

....

....

What did I learn?

....

....

How anxious do I feel afterwards (0–100%)?

....

Do I need to repeat the experiment?

....

....

Do I need to do anything differently next time?

....

....

What am I going to do?

....

....

What am I worried is going to happen?

....

....

How anxious do I feel beforehand? (0–100%)

....

What actually happened?

....

....

Was my prediction correct?

....

....

What did I learn?

....

....

How anxious do I feel afterwards (0–100%)?

....

Do I need to repeat the experiment?

....

....

Do I need to do anything differently next time?

....

....

What am I going to do?

....

....

What am I worried is going to happen?

....

....

How anxious do I feel beforehand? (0–100%)

....

What actually happened?

....

....

Was my prediction correct?

....

....

What did I learn?

....

....

How anxious do I feel afterwards (0–100%)?

....

Do I need to repeat the experiment?

....

....

Do I need to do anything differently next time?

....

....

How to make a self-soothe box

Self-soothe boxes, also referred to as crisis boxes or sensory boxes, are excellent tools to have access to. They are designed to be full of items that help you to get through periods of distress. Try and fill yours with things that cater to each of your five senses. Here are some suggestions of things you could include that might be helpful:

- ❉ **Taste:** Chocolates or mints, or maybe your favourite tea bags

- ❉ **Smell:** Essential oils, nice hand creams or perfume

- ❉ **Touch:** Stress balls, tangles or something soft like a small cuddly toy

- ❉ **Hear:** A prompt card to remind you to access your happy playlist or favourite song

- ❉ **See:** Photos of people you love, motivational quotes, or perhaps some letters of encouragement

It might also be helpful to keep a list of distractions, helplines or apps that you find useful when you are finding things difficult.

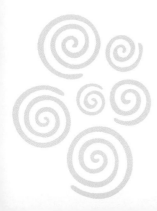

What will go in my self-soothe box?

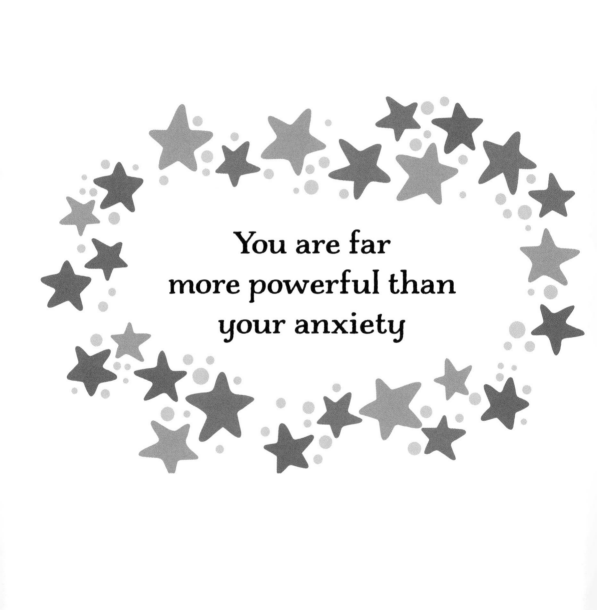

You are far
more powerful than
your anxiety

Communicating with others

When we are struggling with our mental health, we can often end up isolating ourselves from others. This can make it difficult for people to help us, because they either don't know we are feeling this distress, or they aren't sure exactly how to help.

When you are finding things difficult, how could you communicate with people about how you are feeling?

What does my life look like with anxiety?

Anxiety can take up huge amounts of time and energy, and it can ulti-mately get in the way of a lot of other things in our life that are impor-tant to us. Think of this circle as being your life right now. If you were to divide it into a pie chart, how much of that would be controlled by anxiety, and how much would be left for everything else – work, friends, hobbies? For example, maybe anxiety is taking up 80% of your energy and thoughts right now. Doing this exercise can help motivate us to make changes, so that the pie chart of our lives can be full of the things we care about and value.

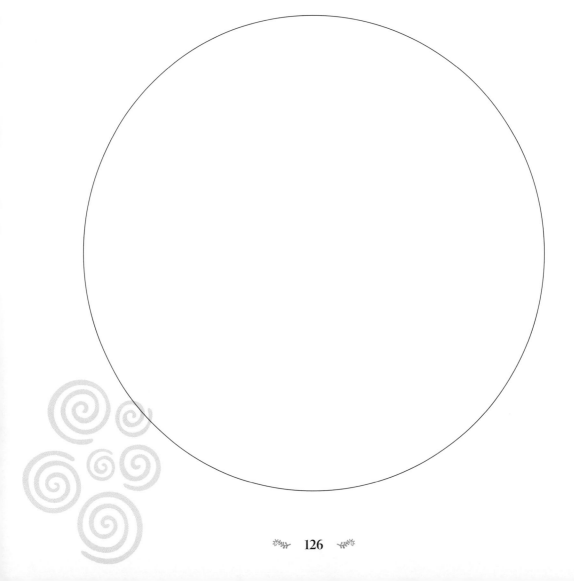

What does my life look like without anxiety?

Now think about what the pie chart of your life would look like if your anxiety difficulties weren't there. How much time would you like to dedicate to things you enjoy? Perhaps you'd like to spend a quarter of your life at work and a lot more of it socializing. Maybe you love studying and want to spend a third of your time doing that. If travelling is your goal, it might take up most of your circle. This is your individual pie chart, and it should align with your own goals and values.

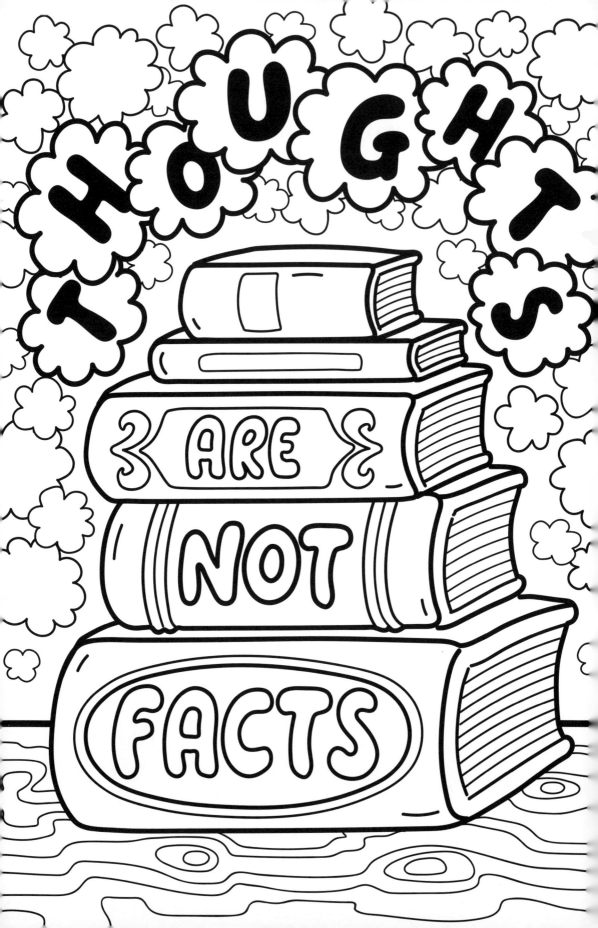

How are you feeling today? Draw or write it out!

What would I say to a friend if they were going through this?

Struggling with anxiety is hugely challenging and can affect not just our lives, but the lives of those around us too. It's easy to be unkind to ourselves as a result of this. Remember, it's not your fault that you have these difficulties. What would you say to a friend if they were going through something similar?

....

....

....

....

....

....

....

....

....

....

....

....

....

....

....

....

....

What would my friends say to me?

What do you think the people in your life who care about you would say to you about your struggles with anxiety?

....
....
....
....
....
....
....
....
....
....
....
....
....
....
....
....
....
....
....
....

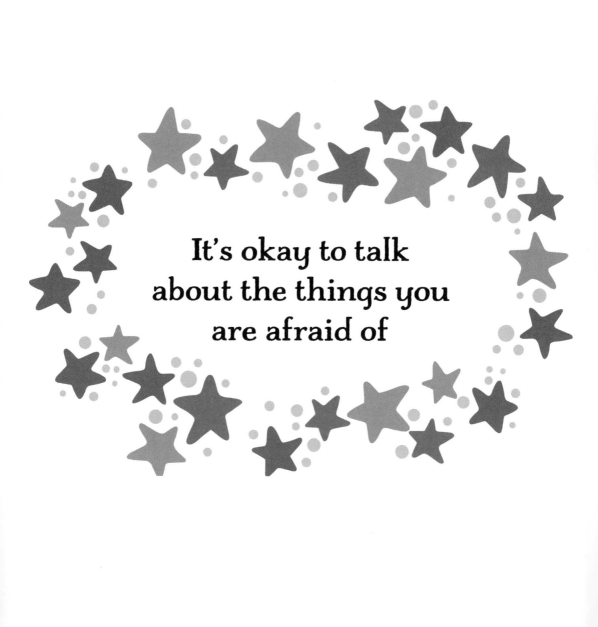

It's okay to talk
about the things you
are afraid of

People who inspire me

We can draw inspiration from lots of different places, but sometimes having people we look up to can be really helpful. Who inspires you to be your best self?

1. ....
....

2. ....
....

3. ....
....

4. ....
....

5. ....
....

6. ....
....

7. ....
....

8. ....
....

9. ....
....

10. ....
....

The future me

We all have a future that isn't ruled by anxiety, but it can be difficult to envisage what that will look like. Have a think about what differences you would notice in the future if you challenged and overcame some of the difficulties you experience with anxiety, compared to what things would be like for you if you don't make any changes.

What will my future look like if I overcome my anxiety?

....

....

....

....

....

....

....

What will my future look like if I don't challenge my anxiety?

....

....

....

....

....

....

....

'I am...' wordsearch

Once you have found the word, repeat the affirmation to yourself out loud.

A	Z	Z	K	Y	B	K	H	E	A	L	I	N	G
P	J	K	W	A	C	F	A	O	N	Y	Q	T	D
L	L	D	J	E	E	W	N	E	F	W	Z	S	O
O	U	U	X	L	Y	Y	K	S	Y	C	D	Q	S
G	S	A	F	E	V	O	W	L	U	F	A	C	L
Z	Y	G	B	P	O	W	E	R	F	U	L	O	K
G	Q	E	K	K	B	B	L	X	M	K	H	B	C
C	A	P	A	B	L	E	G	P	G	B	L	Y	K
A	Z	S	T	R	O	N	G	L	H	U	R	L	A
L	W	K	D	Q	I	A	V	G	M	U	B	F	S
M	I	T	J	W	R	U	U	P	E	L	R	W	A
E	S	R	O	H	M	O	M	J	M	A	A	E	U
N	E	R	G	R	N	B	O	M	B	C	V	C	C
R	G	P	Y	E	Z	H	H	W	S	Y	E	J	P

SAFE   STRONG   CALM
ENOUGH   CAPABLE   HEALING
POWERFUL   GROWING
BRAVE   WISE

Letter writing

What would you say to your anxiety if you could?

....

....

....

....

....

....

....

....

....

....

....

....

....

....

....

....

....

....

....

What are my triggers for increasing my anxiety symptoms?

There are going to be things over the course of your life that might trigger some difficult thoughts or feelings. What might be some triggers for you?

....

....

....

....

....

....

....

....

....

....

....

....

....

....

....

....

....

....

How can I cope with my triggers?

Once we have identified triggers, we can start to notice them more. The world can be a difficult place at times, and sometimes we are going to come across things that trigger us. How can you cope with or manage your triggers?

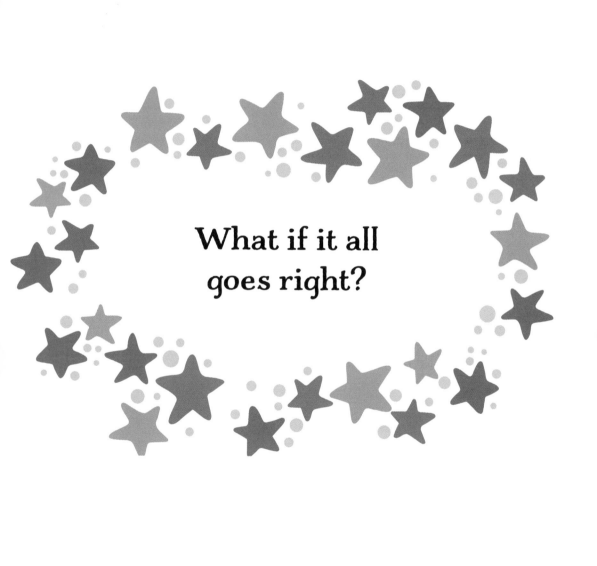

What if it all
goes right?

Letter writing

When you were younger you probably didn't imagine that anxiety would be such a big part of your life. If you could write a letter to your younger self, what would you say?

....
....
....
....
....
....
....
....
....
....
....
....
....
....
....
....
....
....
....

Letter writing

It might be difficult to envision your future without anxiety right now, but it is possible to make changes. If you could write a letter to yourself in the future, what would you say?

....

....

....

....

....

....

....

....

....

....

....

....

....

....

....

....

....

....

....

Early warning signs

It is possible to make a full and sustained recovery from difficulties with anxiety; however, people can often be vulnerable to lapses or relapses in times of stress or uncertainty. What are some early warning signs that things are getting more difficult which you and the people around you should be aware of?

....

....

....

....

....

....

....

....

....

....

....

....

....

....

....

....

....

My traffic lights

Sometimes it can be helpful to think of our progress in terms of a traffic light system: red meaning we need more support, orange meaning we need to be careful and pay more attention to our thoughts and feelings, and green meaning we are well and happy. Have a think about what life looks like for you in each of these zones and what your plan of action would be for each one.

What does my green zone look like?

....

....

....

....

....

....

....

How can I stay in this zone?

....

....

....

....

....

....

....

What does my orange zone look like?

....

....

....

....

....

....

....

How can I get out of this zone?

....

....

....

....

....

....

....

What does my red zone look like?

....

....

....

....

....

....

How can I get out of this zone?

....

....

....

....

....

....

....

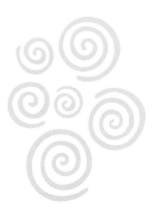

Brain dump

How are you feeling right now? Sometimes getting our thoughts out onto the page can help us to process and make sense of them.

....

....

....

....

....

....

....

....

....

....

....

....

....

....

....

....

....

....

....

....

Managing setbacks

It's important to not only notice when things are starting to get difficult, but also to plan for situations that might result in this happening. What do you think could cause a potential lapse or relapse for you?

What could cause a setback?

....

....

....

....

....

....

....

....

How could I manage this?

....

....

....

....

....

....

....

....

Keeping well

There are lots of things we need to do to keep ourselves on track, some every day and some less often. Have a think about what some of these are for you.

What can I do on a daily basis to keep myself well?

....
....
....
....
....
....
....
....

What can I do on a weekly basis to keep myself well?

....
....
....
....
....
....
....

What do I need to do less often to keep myself well?

. . . .

. . . .

. . . .

. . . .

. . . .

. . . .

. . . .

. . . .

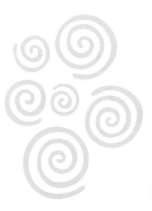

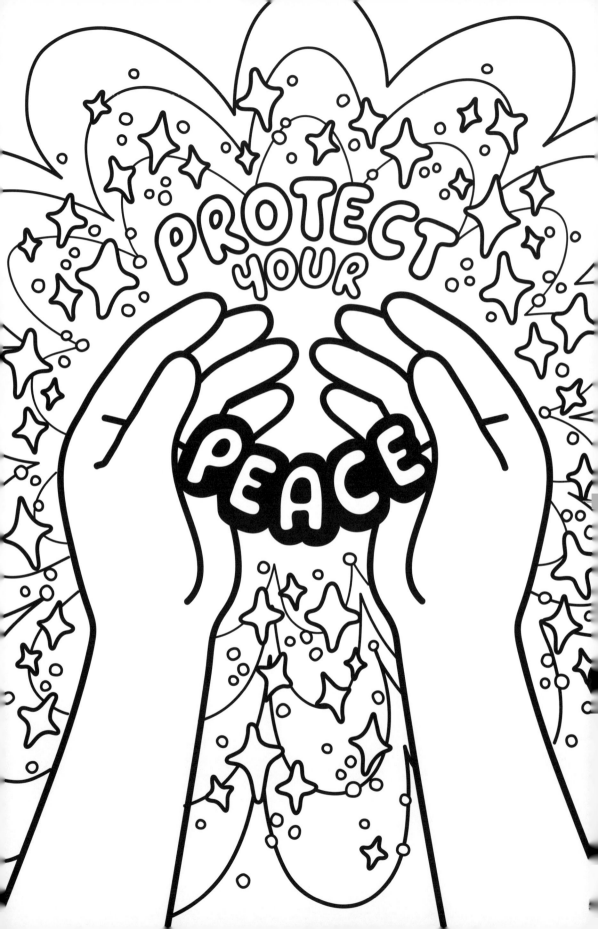

What have I achieved since starting this journal?

I hope that over the time you have been working through this journal, you have been able to start thinking more about ways you can manage and overcome your anxiety. What are some of the things you have achieved, no matter how big or small, since you started using this journal?

....
....
....
....
....
....
....
....
....
....
....
....
....
....
....
....
....
....
....

Congratulations, reader!

You've worked your way through this journal. We hope that you have found some of these exercises useful and that they have got you thinking about ways you can challenge your anxiety and start building a life without it.

There are ways you can continue seeking support, which you will find in the back of this book – these have been recommended by Anneli as resources that have been helpful for her in her own recovery.

We wish you all the luck in the world for your life beyond this journal. Remember, you are more than just your anxiety. Be kind to yourself.

Lots of love, Cara and Anneli

Useful Resources

Websites and helplines

Anxiety UK: www.anxietyuk.org.uk

Anxiety and Depression Association of America: www.adaa.org/understanding-anxiety/generalized-anxiety-disorder-gad/resources

Anxiety Canada: www.anxietycanada.com/downloadables/self-help-strategies-for-gad

Mental Health Foundation: www.mentalhealth.org.uk/explore-mental-health/a-z-topics/anxiety

Mind: www.mind.org.uk/information-support/types-of-mental-health-problems/anxiety-and-panic-attacks/about-anxiety

NHS: www.nhs.uk/mental-health/conditions/generalised-anxiety-disorder/self-help

Young Minds: www.youngminds.org.uk/young-person/mental-health-conditions/anxiety

Books

Staring at the Sun by Irvin D. Yalom (a great book for existential anxiety)

You are a Badass by Jen Sincero

Root and Ritual by Becca Piastrelli

Rewild Yourself by Simon Barnes

How to be Champion by Sarah Millican

Acknowledgements

Cara

I am grateful to my family and friends who are always so supportive of my writing projects. I am especially grateful to Anneli, whose contributions have enriched and added endless value to this book.

I am also thankful to the mental health professionals who have helped me, and also the people I get to support with anxiety, as this has not only helped me to help myself but learn many new ways I can help those I work with.

I hope that I have been able to use all I have learnt from these personal and professional experiences, and created a resource that will be helpful for readers at whatever stage of their journey they are at.

Anneli

Thank you to the mental health community on Twitter. You've been by my side through my recovery journey, and my life is better, easier and less lonely because of you. What a wonderful bunch you are.

A special thank you to L (ily) who has been there for me during some of the scariest times and who has shielded me from a lot of medical Googling. And, of course, to Cara who is one of the most awesome and inspirational people in my life.

My anxiety would be completely unmanageable without the loving support I get from my amazing life partner Macsen who makes everything both calmer and more chaotic in exactly the ways I need. And, of course, my beautiful dog and nap buddy, Douglas Fur, who gives the best cuddles.

To every person who has been brave enough to speak openly about anxiety, to comfort a friend, to ask for support or who has chosen a career in helping people manage their anxiety – you are an absolute rockstar and I hope you know how special and brilliant you really are.

About the Authors

Cara Lisette has struggled with mental illness for much of her life, and through these experiences discovered her love of journalling. She has always seen the value in creativity in fostering good mental health, and this has been endlessly helpful in her own journey towards recovery.

Cara is a registered mental health nurse and qualified psychological therapist. She also runs a successful blog about mental health (www.caras-corner.com) and is active on Twitter (@caralisette) and Instagram (@caralisette), where she talks about her own mental health and recovery in addition to sharing tips and knowledge about mental health overall, from both her personal and professional experiences. She is the author of *The Eating Disorder Recovery Journal, The Bipolar Journal* and *The OCD Recovery Journal,* which are based on her knowledge as a therapist and her lived experience of mental illness.

Anneli Roberts is an artist, writer and mental health advocate who has been living with anxiety and panic attacks since her early teens. She documents her own mental health journey and recovery on Twitter @Pigletish and on her blog pigletish.com, which she started in 2017.

Anneli is passionate about improving the conversation around anxiety and believes reaching out, checking in and talking about the things we're struggling with should all be part of our normal day-to-day conversations.

Anneli was shortlisted for Mind Charity's Digital Champion at the Virgin Media Awards in 2018 and has since made several TV and radio appearances to talk about how anxiety and PTSD have impacted her life.

This journal is one that Anneli wished could have existed when she was first coming to terms with her anxiety, and she thinks it would have been hugely helpful to her in the early days of learning about her condition.

Discover more books from this series...

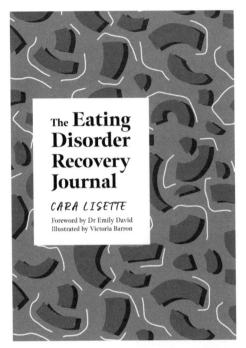

The **Eating Disorder Recovery Journal**

CARA LISETTE

Foreword by Dr Emily David
Illustrated by Victoria Barron

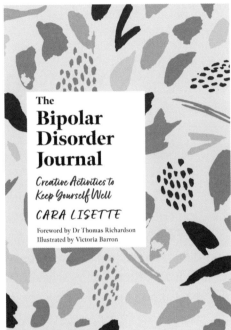

The **Bipolar Disorder Journal**

Creative Activities to Keep Yourself Well

CARA LISETTE

Foreword by Dr Thomas Richardson
Illustrated by Victoria Barron

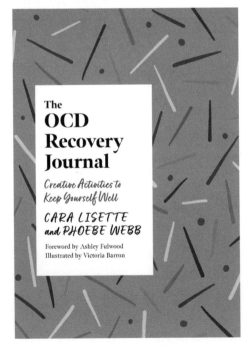

The **OCD Recovery Journal**

Creative Activities to Keep Yourself Well

CARA LISETTE and PHOEBE WEBB

Foreword by Ashley Fulwood
Illustrated by Victoria Barron